By the

Medical Book of Remedies

50 WAYS
TO EASE
FOOT
PAIN

Written by

SUZANNE M. LEVINE

Doctor of Podiatric Medicine

Publications International, Ltd.

All rights reserved under International and Pan American copyright conventions. Copyright © 1994 Publications International, Ltd. All rights reserved. This publication may not be reproduced or quoted in whole or in part by mimeograph or any other printed or electronic means, or for presentation on radio, television, videotape, or film without written permission from: Louis Weber, C.E.O., Publications International, Ltd., 7373 N. Cicero Avenue, Lincolnwood, Illinois 60646. Permission is never granted for commercial purposes. Printed in U.S.A.

Neither the Editors of Consumer Guide® and Publications International, Ltd., nor the author, consultant, or publisher take responsibility for any possible consequences from any treatment, procedure, exercise, dietary modification, action, or application of medication or preparation by any person reading or following the information in this book. This publication does not attempt to replace your physician or other health-care provider. Before undertaking any course of treatment, the publisher, author, and consultant advise you to check with your doctor or other health-care provider.

Author:
Suzanne M. Levine, D.P.M., is a board-certified podiatric surgeon and lecturer who has appeared on the *Oprah Winfrey Show* and has been featured on network television and radio. As a podiatrist in private practice in New York, she has written and published numerous articles and has acted as a resource regarding foot health, beauty, and care to *Vogue, Cosmopolitan,* and other magazines. She is a fellow of the American Academy of Podiatric Sports Medicine and the author of *My Feet Are Killing Me* and *Walk It Off.*

Consultant:
Joseph B. Addante, D.P.M., M.Ed., is an associate in orthopedic surgery (podiatry) and director of the Podiatry Residence Program for Harvard Medical School in Boston. Dr. Addante serves as the chief of podiatry service at the West Roxbury Veterans Administration Medical Center. He is a member of the American Podiatric Medical Association, a diplomate of the American Board of Podiatric Surgery, and a fellow of the American College of Foot Surgeons.

Cover illustration: Leonid Mysakov

FOOT FITNESS AND YOUR HEALTH

FASHION SENSE

INFORMED PATIENT, SMART CONSUMER

INTRODUCTION

If you thought aching feet were just a part of life, have we got some great news for you! In this book, you'll find tips to help you prevent or at least ease the most common types of foot distress.

First, it's important to understand why foot pain is so common. For relatively small body parts, the feet are amazingly complex: Each one contains 26 bones, 56 ligaments, 38 muscles, and an even greater number of nerves and blood vessels. All of those elements are targets for injury, mistreatment, and disease.

The average pair of feet travels up to 70,000 miles in a lifetime. And, though your two feet share the weight of your body when you're standing still, the pressure on each foot increases by 50 percent when you walk and 100 percent when you run.

So it's not surprising that some 87 percent of all Americans suffer from foot ailments at one time or another and that they spend more than $200 million a year on over-the-counter remedies for those problems.

Some foot troubles are hereditary, while others are accidental (nearly six million Americans suffer foot injuries every year). Other foot distress occurs because you've done something unusual: You've started wearing new shoes, you've overdone some activity, or you've ventured into territory where your feet were exposed to infection or other danger. Finally, some foot pain happens only at certain times in life or under certain medical conditions; children's feet and elderly feet in particular need special attention.

While foot trouble affects both men and women, women suffer more pain. Part of the reason is physical: Because women's bodies have a lighter bone structure than men's bodies, the bones in their feet are not as strong and are therefore more susceptible to certain bone problems, including bunions and fractures. Female hormones also affect a woman's foot bones and ligaments. But the main reason women suffer so much foot pain is they're more likely to wear painful, unsupportive shoes.

This book is intended as a handbook. You will find relief strategies for everyday foot discomforts and treatment tips for injuries and other foot dangers. Individuals who have special concerns, especially those who have diabetes or circulation problems, will find information to help them care for their feet. You'll also find groups of remedies designed to help you keep your feet fit and choose footwise footwear.

If you are suffering from a specific problem, you can look it up quickly in the table of contents and turn to the needed information. But we urge you to read the entire book when you get a chance, so you'll be prepared no matter what happens in the future. There are certain foot problems so serious that you should seek a doctor's care immediately; these situations are discussed in remedy 49; *be sure to read this remedy before self-treating any foot problem*. More than anything else, however, this book is designed to give you practical information and suggestions for protecting and treating your feet today, so you can put your best foot forward tomorrow.

1

KNOW YOUR OWN FEET.

Feet are like snowflakes: No two are the same, even those on the same body. Your two feet may actually be different shoe sizes, a situation we'll discuss later in the book. But even if they're evenly matched, they'll be different sizes and different shapes at different times in your life, as your body changes through growth, pregnancy (for women), disease or disability, and aging.

Many foot problems—including bunions, hammertoes, flat feet, gout, even ingrown toenails—are hereditary. And, although greatly influenced by calcium intake, exercise, and hormonal changes, bone strength is partly hereditary. It's also influenced by racial factors. Asians, for example, have less bone mass than whites, and whites have less bone mass than blacks; the greater your bone mass, the less likely you are to develop arthritis or the brittle bones of osteoporosis. One recent study, published in *The New England Journal of Medicine,* found that during puberty—

when hormonal changes spur bone development—the bone density of black girls increases three times more than that of white girls. And when the U.S. Public Health Service conducted a national survey in 1990, it found that blacks experienced 20 percent fewer foot problems overall than whites, although blacks are more likely to suffer from corns, calluses, and flat feet.

Nationality can also influence foot structure: Many Mediterranean people, for instance, have particularly low arches, while many Northern Europeans tend to have high ones. Finally, in some ethnic communities, cultural standards play a role, because they determine what is considered attractive. Members suffer pain from wearing uncomfortable shoes that are simply *de rigueur* in their cultural world.

One of your best precautions against foot pain is to be aware of both the hereditary factors (which you can't change) and the lifestyle and life-stage factors (which you can change or, at least, influence) that determine whether your feet are healthy or hurting.

2

CUSHION AND SOFTEN A TOUGH CALLUS.

A callus is an area where dead skin has accumulated to form a thick, extra-protective patch. Calluses develop on parts of your skin that are exposed to an unusual amount of pressure or friction on a regular basis and therefore need to be tougher than the rest of your skin. Calluses on the feet are common in people who walk around barefoot outdoors, wear shoes that pinch (in which case the calluses develop on the outside of the big and little toes), or wear open-backed shoes (calluses develop under and around the heel). Some calluses on the balls of the feet are caused by shoes that are too loose: The callus develops when the foot consistently rides forward inside the shoe with each step. Other calluses develop on the balls of the feet or just behind the toes because the foot has a low or high arch.

Calluses can begin to hurt if they become too thick. If you have a callus that hurts, try padding your shoe—in the spot where the callus touches it—with a callus pad or moleskin, available in most drugstores. Another solution is to use custom-made orthotics (insoles) that will not only relieve the pressure on the painful callus but also redistribute the abnormal forces causing the callus. Ask your doctor about these.

You can also try soaking your foot in warm water for about 20 minutes, then scrubbing the calloused area with a brush and applying softening cream (if you are diabetic or have circulatory problems, however, see remedies 31 and 32 first); do this at least twice a week. Another great treatment for calluses is remedy 5, which contains a "special recipe" for soft feet. Do not, however, try to cut off a callus.

Intractable plantar keratosis is very deep callus material that develops under the ball of the foot due to a problem with the metatarsal (foot) bone. This condition can be very painful. Treatment usually consists of padding, custom-made insoles, and sometimes surgery to realign the metatarsal bone.

3

CHANGE YOUR SHOES TO CURE A CORN.

Corns are bumps that actually look like kernels of corn. Like calluses, corns develop because of friction and pressure. Corns, however, appear only on or between toes. They develop when toes don't coexist comfortably, either because the toes are not shaped correctly or, most commonly, because they're jammed into shoes that don't fit properly. Corns cause pain not only on the surface of the foot, where the top of the corn rubs against a shoe, for instance, but also inside the toe, where the root of the corn exerts pressure on sensitive nerves. What's worse, the more friction on the corn and the more pain you experience, the faster the corn will grow. Corns can be "hard" or "soft." Soft corns are found between toes, where the moist environment keeps them softer than the hard corns on the tops of toes.

Permanent correction of extremely painful or chronically inflamed corns is usually achieved only with collagen injections or surgery. With most corns, however, the solution is simply a change in footwear—to shoes with a wider toe box or, when possible, to sandals. Some specialists recommend not using drugstore "corn pads," which contain salicylic acid that can burn not just the dead skin of the corn but also normal skin around it. This, in turn, can cause inflammation and/or infection. The other treatments listed here are likely to be effective against corns without risking damage to healthy skin.

If a corn hurts by itself, even when it's not being bothered by shoes, it's likely you've also developed bursitis (see remedy 14), an inflammation of the area around a joint. For temporary relief—while you're looking for those new shoes—try soaking your feet in a solution of warm water and Epsom salts for 20 minutes and then applying moisturizing cream to the offending area (if you have circulatory problems or are diabetic, however, read remedies 31 and 32 first). Don't try to scrape or cut off a corn yourself. You're likely to simply wound yourself, causing bleeding and increased pain and inviting infection.

4

MOISTURIZE DRY SKIN.

Some people suffer dry skin all their lives. Others acquire it as they age and the body begins to lose its natural elasticity and moisture. This change affects the feet as well as the rest of the body. In fact, feet are among the body parts most likely to have dry skin.

Left untreated, dry skin can crack and become painful. This is especially true for the skin on the backs of the heels (which rubs against shoe heels) and under the toes. Xeroderma is a mild dry-skin condition that stems from a seasonal decrease in humidity. It most often affects older people (whose skin naturally has less moisture than that of younger people) during the wintertime. Severe dry-skin conditions include eczema and psoriasis, both of which are rashes that are scabby and very itchy and that can show up all over the body, including the feet. If they occur between toes and cause the skin to crack, they can make walking painful. Chronic dry, cracked skin, especially around the edges of the heel, can even be a warning sign of a thyroid disorder or diabetes.

Take whatever everyday precautions you can to slow this loss of body moisture. For example:

- Avoid wearing shoes without socks or wearing backless shoes, both of which can cause or worsen dry skin.

- Use a humidifier in your home.

- Shower in lukewarm or cool, not hot, water. If you prefer baths, use bath oil, but use caution when getting in or out of the tub.

- Don't bathe too frequently (no more than once a day), since overcleaning the skin robs it of some of its natural moisture.

- Avoid harsh deodorant soaps.

- Soak your feet in water for about 20 minutes; apply moisturizer.

If you suffer from eczema, psoriasis, or another more serious skin condition, see a doctor about what ointments might work best for you.

5

TRY A "SPECIAL RECIPE" FOR SOFT, RELAXED FEET.

Here are some soothing secrets that can be helpful in combatting the problems and discomforts of calluses and dry skin.

To soften skin, try this special recipe once a week:

1. Crush six aspirin tablets and mix them with a tablespoon each of water and lemon juice to make a paste.

2. Apply the paste to callused spots and dry skin on both feet.

3. Place each foot in a plastic bag; wrap a warm towel around each.

4. Sit with your feet wrapped and elevated for ten minutes.

5. Remove the towels and bags, and scrub any rough, dry spots with a pumice stone. The dead skin should now be soft and loose enough to come off.

You can use moisturizing cream in a different version of this routine. Apply the cream right before you go to bed, and then cover your feet with plastic wrap. Sleep with your feet elevated on a pillow, and don't remove the wrap until morning. (Be careful not to wrap the plastic so tightly that it restricts circulation.)

Another home recipe for softening dry skin is to soak your feet in a very dilute solution of water and camomile tea. Afterward, wash your feet with soap and water to remove the tea stains. Then, apply moisturizer.

Of course, any kind of footbath will help to soften dry skin. Just be sure to apply moisturizer immediately after soaking.

A towel wrap can help fight dry skin and relax tired muscles, too. Just wrap each foot in a dry towel, then wrap a towel that has been soaked in hot water around the dry towel. Add two or three layers, alternating dry towels with wet, hot towels; finish with a dry towel. Keep the towels on for 20 minutes. Then, apply moisturizer.

PAMPER A BOTHERSOME BUNION.

A bunion is frequently a form of arthritis, or bone degeneration. It usually takes the form of a bony bump on the outside of your big toe, although bunions can sometimes appear on the top of the big toe joint or even on the little toe (often called a "bunionette"). More than four million Americans have bunions. Most bunions are painful because they're accompanied by bursitis (see remedy 14) and/or because they're so prominent that there's no way to avoid bumping and rubbing them. A bunion may also force your big toe to point inward and rub against the next toe, eventually causing the second toe to become a hammertoe (see remedy 7).

A common myth about bunions is that they're caused by wearing high heels or other shoes that exert pressure on the outside of your big toe. While ill-fitting shoes can certainly make bunions worse, bunions are mostly hereditary. If your parents have bunions, you stand a good chance of having them, too. Bunions tend to come in pairs. In other words, if you have a bunion on your left foot, you'll probably also have one on your right foot.

Here are the best immediate treatments for bunion discomfort:

- Apply ice to the area several times a day.

- Soak the bunioned foot, or feet, in a mixture of one cup vinegar to one gallon warm water.

- Pad the insides of shoes with moleskin or foam rubber cut into a doughnut shape (the hole is for the bunion).

- Switch to shoes with a bigger toe box, or, best of all, wear sandals that leave the bunion area exposed.

In the early stages of bunion pain, a doctor may prescribe orthotics (insoles) and exercises that may stabilize the foot and prevent further development of bunions. For continuing pain, however, you may need bunion surgery, which can often be performed on an outpatient basis.

CUSHION A HAMMERTOE AND GIVE IT SOME SPACE.

Hammertoes are twisted toes that resemble a bird's claw. Hammertoes tend to be hereditary, although they can sometimes occur as the result of an injury to the toe, neurological trauma (such as a stroke), or years of wearing extremely tight-fitting shoes.

Hammertoes are usually hereditary because bunions (see remedy 6) are usually hereditary. A bunion, which appears as a bony bump on the outside of your big toe, may force your big toe inward. This, in turn, forces your second toe, and sometimes even the outer toes, out of shape. This will create hammertoes. The fifth, or little, toes can also become hammertoes if your arches are pronated, or flattened.

Hammertoes hurt when their unusual shape forces them to rub against the inside of a shoe or against the other toes. If the hammertoe is rubbing against the inside of the shoe, a corn (see remedy 3) may develop on the top of the toe.

The best ways to relieve hammertoe discomfort follow:

- Choose shoes that have a lot of room above the toes. This extra room will help accommodate the twisted hammertoe and help prevent the hammertoe from rubbing against the inside of the shoe.

- Pad the hammertoe. This can help protect the hammertoe from excessive friction inside the shoe.

- Whenever possible, wear open-toed sandals or slippers that won't put pressure on your toes.

For a very painful hammertoe, surgery—surgical release of a tight or shortened tendon and/or small-bone removal—may be advised. If your hammertoe is causing continued pain despite the home remedies suggested here, see a podiatrist to discuss the medical options for treatment.

8

STOP PINCHING A PAINFUL NEUROMA.

Morton's neuroma is a noncancerous tumor that results from the thickening of the sheath, or covering, of a nerve. Most neuromas develop between the third and fourth toes when nerves in that area are repeatedly pinched by toe joints or by ill-fitting shoes.

To treat associated pain, burning, and numbness:

- Soak the foot in lukewarm water daily.

- Choose shoes that have a wider toe box.

- Pad the area inside your shoes that corresponds to the site of the neuroma.

A doctor may be able to relieve your neuroma pain for a short period by injecting cortisone into the area. Most neuromas, however, must eventually be surgically excised; otherwise, continued nerve pressure can cause greater and more frequent episodes of pain and numbness.

9

CUT NAILS STRAIGHT ACROSS TO PREVENT AN INGROWN TOENAIL.

Though sometimes ingrown toenails are hereditary, they're most often caused by incorrect nail trimming. They become even more painful when they're squeezed by shoes that are too short and tight. To prevent ingrown nails, trim your nails not in a rounded shape, but straight across the top. In addition, avoid wearing shoes or socks that squeeze your toes together.

An ingrown toenail may cure itself as the nail grows. In the meantime, you can relieve the pain with the steps that follow (if you are diabetic or have poor circulation, however, seek professional attention).

- Switch to longer shoes that have a bigger toe box.

- Soak your foot in a solution of one part povidone iodine to one part water once a day for 20 minutes to reduce the inflammation.

- Trim your nails as best you can. But don't "dig out" a deeply ingrown nail.

- Apply an antiseptic once a day, preferably after a bath or shower. This is especially important, since one of the greatest dangers of ingrown toenails is the possibility of infection.

Your nail cuticle can also become sore as a side effect of an ingrown toenail. If this happens to you, you'll experience redness, swelling, and pain around the cuticle. To reduce the discomfort and inflammation and prevent fungal infection, soak the affected foot in a solution of one part povidone iodine to one part warm water twice a day for about 15 minutes and apply an antiseptic after each soak. Continue until the cuticle is free of pain and back to a normal appearance.

If an ingrown nail is left untreated or is forced too far into the skin by the pressure of shoes, it may not grow out on its own. The only treatment in this situation is to see a doctor, who can numb the toe and remove the offending portion of the nail permanently.

10

INTERVENE IF A NAIL IS INJURED OR INFECTED.

Ingrown toenails are not the only source of nail distress. Often a nail becomes painful due to injury: You've dropped something on it or you've bruised it by stubbing it or banging it repeatedly against the too-tight toe box of your running shoe. In other cases, nails become weak because of poor nutrition (generally, a vitamin C deficiency) or other factors.

Nail discoloration—a "blackened toe-nail"—happens when blood accumulates underneath a nail. Usually the discoloration will go away by itself, although sometimes you may feel pain when the tender toenail pushes against your shoe. If so, place a bandage or piece of tape around the nail to cushion it while it recovers. If your nail doesn't heal by itself, see a doctor, who can numb the toe and drill a small hole in the nail to let the pooled blood out.

If you have naturally brittle nails, which are more easily injured, rub lanolin or petroleum jelly on them every day. If you've jarred a nail and it seems loose or the top appears disconnected from the skin around it, bandage the nail securely for a few weeks (but change the bandage frequently) while the injured part has a chance to grow out and be replaced by strong nail.

Sometimes a bad jolt can cause the nail to separate from the nail bed, loosening at first at the bottom of the nail. This is called onychomadesis. The nail may come completely off. A new nail will grow in, but that can take as long as six months. In the meantime, you must protect the tender toe by covering and padding it to prevent infection and painful contact with shoes.

Another nail condition is onychomycosis, a fungal infection also known as ringworm of the nail. It usually begins at the end of the nail, though the whole nail gradually turns black or brown and becomes thin and flaky. If you develop ringworm, see a doctor. He or she will probably trim your nails very short, try to remove as much of the fungus as possible, and prescribe an antifungal agent.

Then there's onychauxis, a condition common in older people in which the nail has grown extremely thick and has become uncuttable. If this happens to your nail or to the nail of an older person under your care, don't try to cut it yourself; instead, let a doctor file down the nail with a special drill or remove the nail under anesthesia.

Some disorders of the nail are side effects of disease. Infections such as syphilis and tuberculosis affect many body systems, including the nails. Arthritis can produce ridges in your nails. Certain skin conditions, such as psoriasis, can loosen nails and make them brittle.

There are several prescription and over-the-counter products on the market specifically for the treatment of toenail infections and other nail troubles. But most nail problems can be avoided if you follow a simple routine for nail health:

- Trim your toenails straight across the top rather than trying to round them out.

- Wear shoes that don't put pressure on the tops or sides of your toes.

- Make sure that you eat enough foods that are rich in vitamin C.

BE CAUTIOUS IF YOU HAVE PEDICURES.

This often-violent ritual can damage nail cuticles so that they become painfully inflamed and even infected. There are other dangers, too. Some pedicurists use only a cold-sterilization procedure on their instruments and have their customers all dip their feet into a common whirlpool foot-bath. Under these circumstances, you can pick up warts and other foot viruses while you're being "pampered."

If you enjoy pedicures, take your own instruments—nail clipper, files, scissors—with you. If you don't, you should certainly share these concerns with the shop owner and ask what sterilization precautions are taken against such problems. And there's always the option of doing your own soaking, scrubbing, massaging, and painting at home, which may be just as enjoyable!

12

SUPPORT, BUT DON'T FRET ABOUT, FLAT FEET.

"Flat feet" is the ordinary term for feet that are "pronated"—they have very low or no arches, so that when you walk, your entire sole hits the ground. Sometimes this condition is hereditary. In other cases, it's a side effect of something else, such as knock-knee (legs that curve inward at the knee), Achilles tendon tightness, or hormonal or degenerative changes in the body.

Though flat feet have long been a cause of ridicule, arch pronation is actually the fifth most commonly reported foot problem. If you're one of the nearly five million Americans who have flat feet—and yours don't cause you pain—there's no need to do anything to "fix" them. If you do experience pain, however, talk to a doctor about getting orthotics—medically prescribed shoe inserts—that can provide the arch support you need.

DO AWAY WITH WARTS.

Warts are actually benign (noncancerous) tumors; when they occur on the soles of the feet, they are called "plantar warts." Warts are caused by a virus that enters the foot through a cut or crack in the skin. Many warts disappear as mysteriously as they arrived. But not all warts go away on their own, and some can become painful, especially if they are in an area that receives a lot of pressure.

One of the most important elements of treating warts at home is keeping your feet dry. To accomplish this:

- Use over-the-counter foot powder. Sprinkle it onto your feet and into your shoes to absorb moisture.

- Wear absorbent socks. If you find that your feet sweat a great deal, change your socks during the course of the day.

- Wear shoes with uppers made of a porous material, such as leather, that allows air to reach your feet.

- Soak your feet in a tub of warm water that is highly saturated with salt.

- Dry your feet thoroughly after bathing or showering.

Commercial treatments for warts include salicylic-acid pads, ointments, and solutions. If you use these, follow the package directions very carefully to avoid burning the surrounding normal skin. To help protect the surrounding skin when using the ointment or solution form, apply petroleum jelly in a ring around the wart or use a doughnut-shaped pad cut to fit around the wart before applying the medication. Never attempt to cut off a wart. Stubborn warts can be treated by a doctor through laser surgery or by freezing or burning them away.

To help prevent warts, avoid walking barefoot on surfaces where contamination may be lurking, such as public shower stalls; wear thongs in such situations.

SOAK AND CUSHION YOUR FEET TO BEAT BURSITIS.

Bursitis is a painful condition that results when a bursa becomes inflamed. Bursas are fluid-filled sacs positioned around your joints to protect them. While bursitis in the feet can be provoked by wearing ill-fitting shoes, a bursa often becomes swollen and inflamed as the side effect of a corn (see remedy 3), heel spur (see remedy 15), or bunion (see remedy 6).

To help relieve bursitis discomfort:

• Soak your feet in warm water and Epsom salts once a day for 20 minutes.

• Apply ice packs for the same amount of time to reduce swelling.

• Pad the area.

• Wear well-cushioned shoes that fit your feet properly.

If pain persists, see a doctor, who may take an X ray to determine the cause of continuing pain.

TAKE THE PRESSURE OFF A BONE SPUR.

Like a bunion or a hammertoe, a bone spur is generally not preventable, and all you can do about it—short of having corrective surgery—is try to cope with it. A spur is a calcium growth on a bone that exerts pressure on the surrounding tissue and on the skin beyond the tissue. As exotic and awful as the idea of growing a "spur" seems, it's not uncommon: Each year, it happens to about a million Americans. Spurs can grow on various bones in the foot (as well as other bones in the body), but the kind that's most often associated with pain is the heel spur. Because the weight of your whole body presses down on your heel, any pain in that area is intensified and calls for relief. While they can develop in anybody, heel spurs hurt most in heavier people (including pregnant women) and in athletes who repeatedly land hard on their heels in running or jumping.

The best temporary remedy, especially if bursitis (see remedy 14) has also developed around the spur, is to keep from exerting continued pressure on it—stay off the foot and keep it out of shoes as much as you can. Other helpful treatments include applying ice packs to the area and using an over-the-counter painkiller, such as acetaminophen or ibuprofen. When you must wear shoes and walk around, put a foam or felt heel pad (U-shaped in the case of a heel spur) inside your shoe. A doctor may prescribe weight loss, special physiotherapy, injections, orthotics, or anti-inflammatory medication; sometimes a walking cast is also recommended when there is severe pain. And ask your doctor about stretching exercises you can do that will alleviate the pain. But if your bone spur doesn't respond to any treatment or gets worse—if the calcium buildup continues or if there is bleeding inside the foot—you may need surgery.

16

PUT OUT THE FIRE OF BLISTERS AND "BURNING" FEET.

New or ill-fitting shoes are most often the cause of blisters on the feet—those red, burning sores, puffed up and filled with fluid, that appear when shoes rub sensitive skin the wrong way. Blisters can also crop up as the side effect of another problem, such as an itchy infection that you've scratched.

The majority of blisters are preventable if you follow the dictates of common sense: Choose shoes that fit properly and wear cushioning socks. If you seem to get blisters whenever you're "breaking in" new shoes, even when you are wearing socks, you might try going a step or two further. To reduce friction, put petroleum jelly or foot powder directly on the most sensitive spots on your feet, including the backs of your heels, the balls of your feet, and the tops and sides of your toes. Then cushion by inserting moleskin pads in shoes.

Not all feet are structurally alike, and the way your particular feet are made may place extra pressure on weight-bearing areas. Sometimes this pressure will produce blisters, but only during certain activities—for instance, during running but not walking. If you find that you develop blisters in specific areas during certain activities, custom-made insoles may prevent a recurrence (see your podiatrist).

If you have a red, sore area where you think a blister might be developing, cover it with a bandage immediately and keep the bandage on as you wear shoes over the next several days. If you have developed an actual blister, treat it as soon as you can (if you have circulation problems or diabetes, read remedies 31 and 32 first), preferably before a lot of fluid has time to build up inside it. Here's what to do:

1. Thoroughly wash your hands.

2. Clean the blister area with alcohol or an iodine solution.

3. Puncture the blister with a needle you've sterilized by soaking in alcohol.

4. Leave the top on the blister. DO NOT attempt to pull it off. This can cause infection.

5. Apply a topical antiseptic to the blister and the surrounding skin.

6. Cover the area with a bandage or piece of sterile gauze taped into place, and keep it covered for several days.

If your blister doesn't heal or is extremely painful, see a doctor. To prevent future blisters, you should not only switch (or pad) your shoes, but also keep your feet dry and powdered. Excess foot moisture promotes bacterial problems that can lead to peeling and blistering skin. Be especially sure to take these precautions during warm weather, since heat increases body perspiration and foot wetness, or if you are regularly in a place where your feet sweat and/or are exposed to wetness, such as a health club. Don't wear the same pair of shoes (or sneakers) every day.

Uncomfortable, unsupportive shoes—if you walk around in them long enough—will also eventually cause a burning sensation in the soles of your feet. Probably all experienced travelers have at one time or another paid this painful price; many now make their excursions in shoes chosen for comfort and support. (For more information on well-made, supportive walking shoes, see remedy 47.)

Sometimes, however, your feet feel as if they're on fire because they're just plain hot. They're roasting inside shoes that don't "breathe." In other words, the shoes don't allow heat and moisture to escape through the upper or be absorbed by the shoe lining. To keep your shoes from becoming ovens, choose ones with absorbent linings and with uppers made of canvas or other porous material (some leather-topped athletic shoes have little holes in their uppers for just this purpose). You can also have your current shoes relined with a natural, absorbent material.

FIND THE ROOT OF AN ALLERGY OR RASH.

Sometimes one person's feet can react badly to something most other feet don't mind at all. This condition is called contact dermatitis. The offending allergen could be something you've accidentally brushed up against while barefoot. It could also be something you've put on your feet, such as the material of your socks; a new foot powder you're using; or the leather, fabric, or rubber in your shoes.

If you develop a rash or experience itching, think of what's new in your foot's life, eliminate it for a while, and see if the rash disappears. If it doesn't, an over-the-counter antifungal cream may help it go away; follow package directions. (If the symptoms persist or become very painful, see an allergist.) Once the allergy begins to recede, you can help relieve inflammation by soaking your feet in lukewarm water.

There's another possible culprit in the rash category. What you think is an allergy may actually be athlete's foot, a contagious fungal infection that develops between toes or on soles when the foot is exposed to an excessive amount of moisture. Athlete's foot is often acquired by walking around barefoot in wet places, such as swimming pools and health-club showers, where fungal infections spread easily. Most cases respond to over-the-counter antifungal creams, and there are many new topical drugs available that are very effective, including econazole nitrate (1%). Sometimes, special tests are needed to determine what offending organism is causing your particular case of athlete's foot and to prescribe appropriate treatment.

To prevent athlete's foot—as well as the foot wetness that can worsen a case of it—dry your feet and toes thoroughly after showering, wear absorbent socks (and change them often), and don't wear the same shoes day after day. This is especially important for athletes, who should buy two pairs of athletic shoes and switch back and forth between them daily.

DRINK FLUIDS TO CONTROL GOUT.

Gout is a form of arthritis, and there are approximately one million Americans who suffer from this painful condition. Nearly all people with gout have too much uric acid in their blood. Uric acid is normally formed when the body breaks down waste products called purines; the uric acid is dissolved in the blood, passes through the kidneys, and is excreted in the urine. However, if the body makes too much uric acid or if the kidneys are not able to get rid of it fast enough, high levels can accumulate in the blood. Gout generally occurs when the uric-acid level in the blood is so high that crystals of the acid are deposited in the joints, causing the lining of the joints (or synovium) to become inflamed.

Gout attacks can affect joints throughout the body, but they usually affect only one joint at a time. Gout appears most often in the first joint of the big toe.

Heredity may play a role in gout. Taking diuretics, or "water pills," often causes high blood levels of uric acid, because these drugs interfere with the kidneys' ability to remove uric acid. Obesity, overindulgence in alcohol, and eating foods that may raise uric-acid levels (such as brains, kidneys, liver, and sweetbreads) have also been linked to high blood levels of uric acid.

If you suffer an attack, a doctor can prescribe medicine to reduce the swelling and pain. Even if untreated, attacks tend to recede in five to ten days. However, repeated attacks can cause lasting joint damage, so if you suspect you have gout, see a doctor. To help prevent attacks:

- Avoid drinking too much alcohol.

- Talk to your doctor about avoiding certain foods.

- Get your weight under control using a sensible weight-loss program. Avoid crash diets, since they can increase uric-acid levels.

- Drink at least 10 to 12 eight-ounce glasses of water or other nonalcoholic fluid each day to help your body remove uric acid.

APPLY FIRST AID TO FOOT CRAMPS AND ACHING MUSCLES.

Many of us have done it—plunged right into an overambitious exercise program that left our muscles yelping. Foot cramps are one common result when your muscles are not ready for sudden activity. They can also be a sign that your muscles are not getting enough oxygen because your body is becoming dehydrated through perspiration. That's why you should drink plenty of fluids before, during, and after exercise. Sometimes a biomechanical imbalance in feet will cause cramping of shortened muscles; the best prevention in this situation is stretching exercises. Finally, muscle cramping can sometimes be a result of an electrolyte (sodium/potassium) imbalance caused by overuse of diuretics, some of which deplete the body of potassium. Eating bananas, drinking orange juice, or taking potassium supplements can often help in this situation, but be sure to check with your doctor first.

When you do experience cramps, place your feet under running water, starting with cool water and switching to lukewarm. Then give yourself a good foot massage (for instructions, see remedy 43).

Strenuous activity—an unusual amount of walking, running, climbing, or even simply standing—can also hurt the muscles in your foot's arch. The arch is the area of tissue that runs along the bottom of the foot from the heel to the ball. The best remedies include rest and a regimen of ice packs followed a few hours later by heat. Massaging the foot will also help.

You can prevent future cramping and muscle pain by wearing well-made shoes, especially when you walk or run (for tips on choosing athletic shoes, see remedy 47). If you want to begin an exercise program but haven't been very active before, start slowly and increase the intensity of your workouts gradually.

Severe or continuing arch pain can be a sign that you have developed plantar fasciitis (remedy 22) or tendinitis (remedy 21), which are more serious arch problems.

20

REST AND ICE AN ANKLE SPRAIN.

You have sprained your ankle if you've torn tissue—a muscle, tendon, or ligament. Many people confuse a sprain with a strain, which is an uncomfortable condition caused by overstretching these tissues. Sprains are more serious and can make movement very painful. Because small blood vessels in the area rupture as well, the discomfort is often compounded by swelling and tenderness. Sprains are common in athletes, in people who are overweight or double-jointed, and in pregnant women.

In some sprains, tissue is only partially torn, while in others the rupture is more severe. Pain is a good indicator of the severity of the injury. Fortunately, most tears will heal on their own if cared for properly. If you suspect anything more than a mild strain, have the ankle checked by a physician. To care for a sprained ankle, take the following steps, unless your physician directs you otherwise:

- Rest the foot for a day or two, keeping it elevated.

- Apply ice packs for 15 minutes once every hour over the first 24-hour period or until swelling subsides.

- Use an elastic bandage that will compress the ankle. (However, if you are diabetic or have circulation problems, you should not use elastic bandages without a doctor's approval.)

- When you can do so without great pain, gently exercise the ankle by slowly rotating and flexing your foot.

Even after your sprain heals, the ankle will be more susceptible to additional strains and sprains. To prevent reinjury, wear shoes that provide good support in the ankle area, particularly when you're playing sports. You might also want to tape the ankle during athletic activity. If you do sustain repeated lateral ankle sprains, you may need to wear custom-made orthotics or even have surgery.

21

ALLOW HURT TENDONS TO HEAL THOROUGHLY.

Tendons are the "bridges" that connect muscles to bones all over your body, including in your feet and ankles. Tendinitis is the inflammation, stiffness, and swelling that result when a tendon is strained or torn. You can experience this problem in tendons anywhere in the foot, including those within the arch along the bottom of the foot. But one of the most common—and painful—spots for tendinitis is in the Achilles tendon (actually a group of tendons), which connects the muscles and bones of your lower leg to those of your foot. (It is named for the Greek hero whose only vulnerable spot was the back of his heel.)

Achilles tendinitis is an injury often associated with dancers, runners, and high-impact aerobic devotees—all people who place repeated and great stress on the Achilles tendon. Other sufferers include women who are accustomed to wearing high heels and then suddenly switch to flats. In this case, the tendon is simply not used to being stretched in this new way and becomes sore and swollen.

If the tendon is only overstretched, it should heal within a day or two with a treatment of ice packs, elevation, and rest, similar to the healing routine for ankle sprains. After the first 24 hours, alternate ice packs with heat to help reduce the inflammation that often accompanies tendinitis. When you must be on your feet, put inserts inside your shoes or in some other way cushion the affected area. Wear shoes with a moderate heel rather than flats to lessen the pull on sore tendons. Aspirin or another anti-inflammatory drug can relieve some of the discomfort of mild tendinitis.

Cases of tendinitis in which the tendon is torn partially or completely away from the bone can be quite serious and require a doctor's care, physical therapy, and sometimes even surgery. If surgery is not required, your doctor may still want to give you medication that will reduce swelling and put your foot in a cast to immobilize the area of injury. Whatever treatment is recommended, you're likely to spend several months recovering from the problem.

The best course of "treatment" for this disabling and all-too-common injury is prevention. And it's simple: Stretch. You must prepare your Achilles tendon and other foot tendons for any new activity in which they will be pulled to their full length. If you're a runner or a dancer, definitely do leg and foot stretches before and after your exercise routine. Also wear athletic shoes with a raised heel and with plenty of cushioning and support in the heel, arch, and toe areas. Walkers should take the same precautions; mild tendinitis can develop in the feet of walkers who don't warm up or those who wear very flat walking shoes without heel and arch cushioning. But even if you don't follow any "official" fitness program, stretching exercises (including those in remedy 38) are a good idea and are very easy to do.

22

REST AND APPLY ICE FOR BADLY DAMAGED ARCHES.

The medical term for the tissue along the arch of your foot, starting behind your toes and extending back to the heel, is the plantar fascia. You have plantar fasciitis if that tissue is badly overstretched or partially or fully ruptured. The cause is too much pressure exerted on the arches, and, although common in athletes, the condition can happen because you went hiking or climbing, you were lifting heavy objects, or you simply walked too far too vigorously. Pregnancy places extra strain on the arches due to the additional body weight and the effect of hormones on muscles and ligaments (see remedy 33); if that strain is severe enough, it can not only stretch but tear the plantar fascia. No matter what the cause of your problem, however, the end result is the same: foot pronation—a temporary case of "flat feet"—and pain.

The best treatment: Apply ice packs, followed by heat (to reduce inflammation), to the area for 20 minutes once a day. Rest is also essential. You will have to avoid any activity—in some cases, even standing or walking—that would increase the tear until the tissue heals on its own (this can sometimes take up to six weeks). With strains and less severe tears, you may be able to walk on the foot with arch-support shoe inserts. You'll need to see your doctor for more permanent arch support. A doctor can also provide immediate relief from the pain of plantar fasciitis by giving you a local cortisone injection or prescribing anti-inflammatory medication.

Once the plantar fascia is healed, prevent a repeat injury by:

- choosing shoes, especially athletic shoes, that provide good arch and heel support

- avoiding activities you're not accustomed to that place a lot of stress on the foot

- doing stretching exercises (see remedy 38) to strengthen the muscles and ligaments of your feet.

23

WATCH OUT FOR WHAT'S ON THE GROUND.

Few of us made it through childhood without a painfully itchy, exasperating case of poison ivy, poison oak, or poison sumac. Though this is a danger you should caution your own children about, you can still succumb in adulthood. To avoid getting a rash, learn to recognize and avoid the plants. Poison plants are one good argument for wearing socks and closed shoes outdoors; since many people won't do that in the summertime, however, knowledge and caution are your best defense. If you *do* have a rash reaction—red, itchy patches on the skin—wash the area as soon as possible with soap and water and apply calamine lotion to relieve the itching. Try not to scratch. Time is the only real "cure."

While most of us know to protect ourselves from dangers like poison ivy, few of us give much thought to the ground beneath our feet. And yet it's an important factor in what our feet experience outdoors. If you do any kind of activity that involves movement—walking, running, jumping, or playing a sport—try to do it on a surface that's least likely to jolt feet and ankles or to cause burning soles. Concrete is the worst surface for any such activity because it's inflexible, and every time you land on it, your foot and leg get quite a jolt. If you walk or run regularly, do so on a path of packed dirt, if possible; this type of surface is softer than concrete but not as unstable as gravel or grass (uneven surfaces that can cause you to turn your ankle). Another great choice is packed-down sand, the kind you find on a beach just at the water's edge. Soft, loose sand is the best surface for jumping sports like volleyball. Clay is a better surface for tennis than cement; be especially careful about tripping if you're playing on grass.

24

CLEAN AND COVER A CUT.

Cuts are among the most common foot injuries, since our feet meet with so many surfaces that can contain sharp objects. With a minor cut, wash the area and apply hydrogen peroxide or a topical antiseptic. Then cover the cut with a bandage or sterile gauze or cloth. Minor cuts can take up to ten minutes to stop bleeding; applying pressure to the cut can help stop the bleeding. Most minor cuts will heal on their own if kept clean and covered.

If the cut is deep and blood is spurting out, don't worry about cleaning the area—just cover it as best you can and apply pressure. (If it is a puncture wound, however, see remedy 25.) If you have clean bandaging material handy, use that, but if you don't, wrap an article of clothing around the foot, or even use your hand until someone can bring you a substitute covering. If blood soaks through the first layer of bandage, don't remove it (pulling it up will undo whatever clotting has occurred); just add a second layer.

Even after covering a wound, continue to apply pressure with your hand. If someone is with you, ask him or her to do this while you lie down, with your foot propped up above the level of your heart; if you're alone, try to elevate the foot while applying pressure. By elevating a wound, you slow the flow of blood to that part of the body. This is especially important for the feet, since they are the lowest part of your body.

If you suffer anything other than a superficial cut, see a doctor. A culture and sensitivity test may be required, or you may need antibiotics. Sometimes a tetanus injection is necessary if the wound is particularly deep; if there is inflammation, the wound may need to be drained. If the layer of fat beneath the skin is visible, stitches may be required.

25

DON'T CLEAN OR APPLY PRESSURE IF AN OBJECT HAS PUNCTURED THE SKIN.

If the injury is a puncture wound, seek medical attention, even if the wound stops bleeding or seems minor. You may need a tetanus shot. (Many people think you need a tetanus shot only if you step on a rusty nail. Not so! You can develop tetanus or other infection from all sorts of contaminated items.) If a foreign body remains embedded in your foot, do not try to pull it out; you may widen the wound or, even worse, cause the object to injure a nerve or blood vessel. Avoid applying antiseptics or any bandage that will press the object farther into the flesh. Instead, cover the wound area loosely with a sterile cloth or gauze that will help blood begin to clot. Then get to a doctor or hospital emergency room.

26

KNOW HOW TO TELL IF YOU'VE BROKEN A BONE.

When you break a bone in your foot or ankle, sometimes you know it right away: You feel the sudden and tremendous pain, and you may even hear the bone snap. In other cases, you know you've hurt yourself, but you're not sure if you've broken anything. Look for these signs: You can't move the ankle or foot (or a particular toe), or you can do so only with great pain; the area is painful when you touch it with a finger; the area is swollen or bluish or both. If you're still not sure, play it safe and treat the injury as if it were a broken bone: Immobilize the foot (or ankle)—for instructions on immobilizing a bone that you suspect is broken, see remedy 27—and go to the emergency room.

27

PERFORM ONLY EMERGENCY FIRST AID ON A BROKEN FOOT OR TOE.

If you know or suspect you have a broken bone, carefully remove the shoe and sock and then immobilize the foot, ankle, and lower leg. One way to do this is to splint the entire lower leg, using a board, straight sticks, or even a thick magazine. Place padding (towels or clothes) between the leg and the splint, then tie the splint in place with rope, cloth, or a belt. Tie tightly enough to hold the splint in place but not so tightly that circulation is restricted; do not tie directly over the break. Another way to splint a broken foot or ankle is to gently slip a pillow or folded blanket underneath it, curve it up around the foot and ankle, and tie it in place, creating a circular "cast."

Elevation of the foot helps stop swelling and bleeding, but don't move the foot to elevate it. Instead, if you are being assisted by someone else, lie down on your back, thus "raising" your foot's position in relation to your heart. Unless there is no other way for you to get help, don't hop around on the opposite foot.

If the injury that broke the bone also caused cuts on the foot, stop the bleeding in the ways described in remedy 24. If a bone is protruding from the foot, treat it the same way you would a foreign body in the foot (see remedy 25). Once you've immobilized the foot and stopped the bleeding, get to a hospital emergency room. It's likely that your broken bone will need to be set and placed in a cast. If it's a toe that's broken, it may heal with the help of shoe cutouts or special padding inside your shoes. Wherever the fracture site, however, it's important that you get X rays so a doctor can determine if the broken bones are in proper alignment to heal.

28

STOP OR CHANGE YOUR EXERCISE ROUTINE TO HEAL A STRESS FRACTURE.

Repeated force on a bone or group of bones can cause them to sustain hairline cracks called stress fractures. Most occur in the metatarsal bones, the bones in the front of the foot that attach to your toes. Weakened muscles can exert enough pressure on foot bones to cause a stress fracture; so can gaining a lot of weight over a short period of time.

If you sustain a stress fracture, you'll feel a nagging pain as you walk or run; the area will also hurt if you press on it from above or below with your finger. Because stress fractures are so slight, they heal on their own. But while that process is occurring—it can take weeks—you may have to put a halt to sports or exercise routines. (To keep up your fitness level, temporarily substitute another fitness activity that doesn't put pressure on the feet, such as swimming.) For relief from pain, apply ice packs to the area and take aspirin or ibuprofen.

To prevent stress fractures, wear shoes that provide sufficient padding and support when you walk, run, dance, or perform any other activities that put stress on the bones of the foot. Another precaution is to do such activities on surfaces that "give" (in other words, surfaces that are not inflexible like concrete), such as packed dirt, sand, or rubber matting; this lessens the sharpness of the impact on foot bones every time you step, stride, or bounce.

The stronger your bones are, the less likely you are to suffer from stress fractures. So follow the same advice given in remedy 35 for preventing bone degeneration: Make sure you get plenty of calcium and vitamin D in your diet. Vitamin D, which helps the body assimilate calcium, can be obtained from fortified milk or by getting 20 minutes of sunshine three times a week. If you're a woman past menopause, talk to your doctor about taking calcium supplements and beginning estrogen-replacement therapy. Orthotic therapy may also be indicated.

SOOTHE (AND PREVENT) SUNBURNED FEET.

Sunburn can be especially painful on the tops of feet and toes because skin is so tender there. You experience the same symptoms you do with any burn: pain, redness, swelling, and eventual peeling or blistering. To treat the pain, run cold water over your feet (or soak in it) and apply a cream or lotion that contains aloe, a plant substance that helps heal burns. To prevent future sunburn, wear sunscreen with a sun protection factor—SPF—of 15 or higher.

Note for men and women of color: Do not expose scars or the site of a surgical incision to sunlight; the increased melanin in the skin in combination with the sun will cause hyperpigmentation. If this does occur, use a bleaching cream that contains hydroquinone. For serious hyperpigmentation, see a doctor.

GRADUALLY REWARM FROSTBITTEN TOES OR FEET.

When extremities are exposed to sub-freezing temperatures for too long, ice crystals can actually form in the fluids inside skin and tissue. Frostbite warning signs include numbness (or tingling) followed by pain and skin that turns first red and tender, then white and hard. If you do experience these warning signs, get indoors as soon as possible, carefully remove shoes and socks, and slowly place your feet in lukewarm—not hot—water. If you can't get to water, place sterile padding between frostbitten toes and wrap your feet in blankets. Don't put your feet on top of a stove or radiator: If they're numb, you might not realize you're being burned. Also, do not rub frostbitten skin. As feeling gradually returns, slowly wiggle your toes. If pain continues, go to a hospital emergency room.

HELP BLOOD FLOW TO YOUR FEET, ESPECIALLY IF YOU HAVE POOR CIRCULATION.

Circulation problems are often associated with older feet, but the fact is that anyone can have such problems. Everyday circumstances can restrict blood flow: when feet get cold outdoors or in cold water; when shoes, stockings, or undergarments are too tight; even when you've sat too long with your legs crossed. Smoking reduces circulation to all parts of the body, as does drinking too much coffee or caffeinated soda (both nicotine and caffeine constrict blood vessels). And if you are under severe stress, your nerves can constrict your small blood vessels, lessening their ability to carry blood. (Some nervous brides and grooms really do have "cold feet"!)

Other people have ongoing medical conditions, such as diabetes (remedy 32), that cause sluggish circulation. Some women experience a condition called Raynaud's phenomenon, which is a minor circulation problem, often triggered by cold weather, that causes hands and feet to occasionally feel cold or even numb. This problem is not as serious as Raynaud's disease, in which the arteries lose their ability to dilate (open). If you suffer from either condition, you should be under a doctor's care.

When there's not enough blood flowing to your feet, you may experience tingling, numbness, cramping, and discoloration of the skin and toenails. To increase circulation, wear comfortable, roomy shoes and avoid constricting socks. A warm footbath can help increase circulation, as can massage. Perhaps the best "cure" of all for sluggish circulation is to get your feet moving, since activity promotes blood flow. Try not to sit for long stretches of time; if you must, periodically flex your feet and wiggle your toes (for other suggestions, see remedy 37). A moderate exercise program, such as walking, will improve circulation, not just in your feet but throughout your whole body. If you have a chronic circulation problem, medication may be necessary, and a doctor may want to test your blood flow using special equipment.

32

PROTECT DIABETIC FEET.

For most of us, a cut or blister is an annoying but relatively minor foot problem. For a diabetic, these "little" wounds can have serious consequences. Diabetics' feet are at two general disadvantages that can lead to specific, serious foot problems. A loss of feeling in the foot, called neuropathy, can prevent diabetics from feeling the small aches and pains that normally signal to us that we've been cut or bruised. As a result, minor problems can go unnoticed and untreated, and infection may develop.

Diabetics also have poor circulation, a problem that affects the feet more than any other body part because the feet are farthest from the heart. Poor circulation produces the problems discussed in remedy 31: tingling, cramps, and brittle and discolored toenails. It also slows healing of wounds. If you are diabetic:

- Inspect your feet frequently and carefully, checking for small cuts, cracking skin, blisters, and other spots that will invite infection. If your vision or flexibility is impaired, have someone inspect your feet for you. If you have sores and develop a fever, see a doctor at once. Likewise, if you notice a cut, crack, blister, or corn on your foot, don't try to treat it yourself; go straight to a doctor.

- Avoid walking barefoot; wear socks, even with sandals, to help prevent blisters and calluses that can crack.

- Choose socks that don't restrict blood flow, and choose shoes that provide good cushioning and support, especially in the arch area.

- Bathe your feet often in lukewarm water using mild soap. Dry your feet thoroughly after bathing and use moisturizer.

- Talk to your doctor about trimming your nails.

- Do not smoke, since smoking further restricts blood flow.

- With your doctor's consent, start a program of regular physical activity, such as walking.

33

PAMPER YOUR FEET DURING PREGNANCY.

Feet ache during pregnancy partly because of the greater amount of weight they're carrying and the way that this burden is distributed. Because almost all of the new weight is in one place, your body's natural center of gravity is thrown out of whack. The result is that many ligaments and muscles throughout your body—including those in the feet—are suddenly put under strain and pressure that they don't normally receive.

The problem is exacerbated by the fact that, during pregnancy, hormonal changes send signals to your ligaments, telling them to relax. This happens so that your stomach will stretch to hold your baby. The problem is that all your ligaments relax. When those in the feet and ankles "sag," there are several consequences: Foot fatigue sets in more quickly; you're more susceptible to spraining or twisting your ankles; and you have a good chance of developing the calluses and heel pain that can result from arch problems. The hormonal changes happening throughout your body also make your skin drier, increasing flaking and cracking of the skin on your feet. And the fact that blood circulates less efficiently during pregnancy adds to swelling of the feet and ankles.

The good news is that these foot woes will disappear after your baby is born. Until then, the following tips may help ease the burden on your feet:

- Even healthy feet are usually uncomfortable during pregnancy, but if you have problems that would simply make matters worse—corns, calluses, a heel spur, arch pain—take care of them during the early stages of your pregnancy. If you don't, the swelling and added weight of pregnancy will put enough extra pressure on those problems to turn them from sources of discomfort into sources of real pain.

- Wear low-heeled shoes that provide good arch support and cushioning throughout the shoe. Well-constructed shoes not only alleviate foot aches but also help you maintain your balance, preventing ankle sprains. Wear support hose designed for pregnant women, and avoid tight-fitting socks and undergarments that restrict circulation. When you are at home, switch to comfortable slippers that have good traction on the bottoms but also stretch to conform to the shape of your foot.

- To reduce swelling, soak your feet in cool (but not cold) water. Then massage them, or if it's hard or uncomfortable for you to reach your feet, have someone else massage them (see remedy 43 for instructions on foot massage).

- If foot and ankle swelling becomes painful or makes it hard for you to get around, see a doctor about getting cus-tom-made shoe inserts that will boost the strength of your ligaments.

- If you have never been much of an ath-lete, don't start any ambitious fitness program during pregnancy. But if you've always exercised, there's no reason you shouldn't continue it, under your doctor's supervision. Walking is a particularly good exercise for pregnant women. It's not as hard on sensitive ankles and feet as running and other sports, and yet it helps strengthen foot muscles and ligaments, increase circulation, relieve back pain, and even prevent varicose veins. Since your feet are probably already swollen, however, try to avoid walking outdoors on humid days. And decrease the difficulty of your routine during the second and third trimesters.

- If you feel too tired or too heavy to keep up with your usual workout, you can still keep your feet moving with the foot "energizers" in remedy 37.

- Put your feet up whenever you get the chance. This will reduce swelling and lessen stress on your soles and heels.

- Since skin gets drier during pregnancy, apply moisturizing creams and lotions to your feet (and the rest of your skin), especially after bathing or showering.

WATCH FOR PROBLEMS IN CHILDREN'S FEET.

Children's feet have few of the same kinds of aches and injuries adult feet do, although in many ways they are more susceptible to pain because they're so tender. Among the most common concerns are:

- Warmth: Cold feet can chill a baby all over, decreasing circulation and hastening colds and other illnesses. When you take your baby outdoors (except on hot summer days), put shoes or very warm booties on the baby's feet. Indoors, if temperatures are cool in the winter or your house has a draft, protect your baby with socks or booties or a one-piece outfit that covers the feet.

- Support: Young children haven't had much time to develop the strong foot and ankle muscles that prevent strains or the calluses that protect skin. Therefore, children's shoes should have soft upper material and plenty of cushioning inside. They'll also need plenty of traction on the outer sole to prevent slipping. Well-made shoes also help toddlers maintain their balance.

- Foot growth: Children grow out of shoes rapidly. You need to make sure the shoes they're wearing don't pinch or rub their feet or prevent the proper growth of their feet and toes. Check the fit of your child's shoes every few weeks. Ask your baby's doctor if you're not sure how to do this.

- Nighttime pain: Children between the ages of two and five years often experience severe leg cramps at night. Although doctors once called these "growing pains," we now know that there are reasons—controllable reasons—for this phenomenon. The reasons include fatigue, foot or leg strain, low temperature in the home at night, or poor blood circulation that results from the child's sleeping position. To relieve the pain, massage the cramped area. Also, try to maintain an even temperature in the child's bedroom during the night.

- Rashes and warts: Children often run around barefoot and may be exposed to infectious foot diseases. Children are more likely than adults to suffer from athlete's foot (remedy 17) and plantar warts (remedy 13). Excess moisture can worsen a rash, so make sure your child wears absorbent socks, and dry your child's feet thoroughly after baths.

- Signs of future trouble: Babies are born with flat feet, but by age four or so, the feet should have developed arches. If your child's foot remains flat or seems to have an unusually high arch, see a doctor now. Getting medical care at this stage could prevent years of pain and more serious treatment.

- Sports: Once children begin participating in sports, see that they wear well-made sneakers or athletic shoes that are appropriate to their particular sports. (Follow the same guidelines given for adult athletes in remedy 47.)

- Deformities: The bad news about foot deformities—birth defects of the feet—is that they must be treated as quickly and completely as possible, and sometimes that means surgery. The good news is that many problems that seem terrible at first—such as club (inturned) foot or webbed toes—can be permanently corrected with consistent use of casts, special pads, braces, or special shoes in the early years. Overlapping toes, a not-uncommon problem in infants, can be taped so that they are "trained" to grow straight. Metatarsus adductus—an intoeing gait due to the position of the metatarsal bones—can be corrected with orthopedic shoes, exercises, and orthotic therapy. The important thing is to talk with your child's pediatrician and find a podiatrist as soon as possible after your baby's birth, since the sooner deformities receive medical attention, the greater the chances of complete correction and less pain throughout your child's life.

35

PRESERVE BONE MASS.

Foot aches are often rooted in, or related to, changes taking place in the rest of the body. Osteoarthritis—the form of arthritis associated with the degeneration of bone and cartilage as we age—affects the joints of the feet just as it affects joints in the hands and elsewhere. (Younger people can also suffer a form of the disease called rheumatoid arthritis.) Many of the more than 75 million arthritis sufferers in America have benefited from exercising moderately, increasing levels of calcium and iron in their diets, and taking over-the-counter oral medicines, including aspirin. The most common kind of relief, however, is prescribed medication.

Older feet also face the even greater danger of fracture when a condition called osteoporosis is present. Osteoporosis is the gradual loss of bone mass that occurs in some 20 million elderly Americans, most of them women. Women are more often affected, partly because they have less bone mass to begin with, but also because the female hormone estrogen plays a role in bone strength in women. After menopause, a woman's body produces much less estrogen. Some studies have shown that certain factors—including smoking and alcoholism—can speed the onset of osteoporosis; heredity also plays a role.

The best precaution against developing osteoporosis is to get enough calcium in your diet (and, if necessary, through supplements), since calcium plays an important role in bone strength. You'll also need to be sure you get enough vitamin D—either through fortified foods or sun exposure—to help your body assimilate the calcium. Many doctors recommend that postmenopausal women also receive estrogen-replacement therapy. Moderate but regular weight-bearing exercise is also important, as demonstrated in a study done at Washington University in St. Louis. In the study, healthy women over age 55 walked an hour a day at least four days a week for about a year. This program of exercise appeared to do more than prevent the loss of bone; in most of the women, bone mass actually increased by six to eight percent.

36

GUARD AGAINST PROBLEMS OF OLDER FEET.

Many foot troubles get worse over time, especially if they've never been treated. It stands to reason, then, that older people would be likely to have more of these maladies than the rest of the population and would have more severe cases. Toenail problems and bothersome calluses are particularly common among older people.

To soften calluses, pad your shoes in the callus area, soak your feet frequently, gently use a pumice stone on the callus after bathing, and follow the instructions for the "special recipe" treatment in remedy 5. If your calluses cause you intense pain, see a doctor who can "shave" away the buildup of dead skin.

To prevent thickened and ingrown toenails—very common problems among older people—trim nails regularly (straight across the top); wear shoes with comfortable, wide toe boxes; keep nails clean; and use foot powders that will help keep your feet dry and cut down on fungal infections.

If your nails have become so thick that you can't cut them yourself, go to a doctor to have them cut. Letting them grow will only increase your pain and your chances of developing an infection.

It's inevitable that as you age, your skin will lose some of its elasticity and moisture. For tips on treating dry skin on your feet, particularly when it causes painful problems, see remedy 4. Finally, aging causes you to lose fat, and a thinning of the "fat pads" on the bottoms of your feet will cause sole pain. Neuromuscular or collagen (connective-tissue) diseases also contribute to thinning of fat pads. Custom-made insoles will help cushion the foot inside shoes, but if you continue to experience pain, be sure to see a doctor. He or she may recommend collagen injections or even fat replacement, a still-experimental procedure in which fat is surgically moved from another part of the body to the balls of the feet.

37

RE-ENERGIZE YOUR FEET THROUGHOUT THE DAY.

During the course of a day, your feet, like the rest of your body, gradually lose steam. But you can re-energize them even when you're seated at a desk, at home in front of the television, in class, or on an airplane, train, or bus. In any of these situations, you can do at least one, if not all, of the following pick-me-ups designed especially for feet that do not get to move around much throughout the day. Each of these exercises should be done while you are seated.

- **Foot Relaxer:** Start by relaxing and loosening your foot muscles and joints by shaking them (the same way you'd shake out cramped muscles in your fingers and hands). Then wiggle your toes, first on one foot, then the other.

- **Foot Press:** With your feet on the floor, take your shoes off and place one foot on top of the other. Press the top one down while pulling up with the bottom foot— but don't let your feet separate.

- **Toe Tap:** With your feet on the floor, tap your toes, or pretend that you're pressing down on a pedal, first with one foot, then with the other.

- **Toe Writing:** With your feet on the floor and your shoes off, use your toes to "write" the letters of the alphabet, from A to Z, on the floor.

- **Toe Grip:** With your feet on the floor and your shoes off, try picking up a pencil or pen with your toes. Or try picking up a marble (if you happen to have one lying around).

- **Page Rippler:** With your feet on the floor and your shoes off, place a phone book under your feet, with its binding facing your body. Curl your toes over the far edge and try to ripple the pages.

Once you have revitalized your feet with these seated exercises, you might want to massage your feet a bit. It's a great way to cap off your mini foot workout. See remedy 43 for tips on giving yourself an expert foot massage. More exercises follow:

- **Roller Massage:** If you're sitting at home with your shoes off, place a rolling pin under one foot. Roll back and forth on the pin with that foot; then do the same with the other foot. This is a way of giving yourself a foot massage without pulling your feet into your lap or getting down on the floor. If you like this, you might even take a rolling pin to the office; then, several times throughout the day, take your shoes off and "roll" the tension out of your feet. This "roller massage" will also work with a tall, narrow bottle. Some people use smaller "rollers" including golf balls and even marbles.

- **Flex and Point:** Try this at home or at the office if there's a way you can prop your legs up so that they're facing straight out in front of you and are parallel to the floor. (In the office, you might prop them on a high stool or another chair; if you're sitting on the couch at home, use the coffee table.) Point your toes forward, like a ballerina pointing her extended foot, and hold that position for 15 seconds. Then relax your toes and reposition your feet so that your toes are pointing toward the ceiling. Repeat this routine—flex and point ahead of you, then relax and point to the ceiling—ten times.

- **Curl and Turn:** With your legs propped up in front of you and parallel to the floor, curl your toes, and then (keeping your heels on the surface where they're propped) turn your feet inward. Hold this position for five seconds. Then allow your toes and feet to return to their former, relaxed position.

- **Purse Lift** [for women]: With your back pressed straight against the back of the chair, drape the strap of your purse over one foot. Keeping your knee bent, raise your foot until the purse hangs suspended in the air. Hold that position as long as you can, then lower your foot. Switch the purse to the other foot and repeat the exercise.

38

REGULARLY STRETCH FOOT AND LEG MUSCLES.

The muscles in your feet have a close relationship with those in your legs: Pain in the leg muscles makes it hard for foot muscles to do their job (comfortably), and vice versa. Also, many stretching exercises benefit both the feet and the lower legs. Rochelle Rice Cutro, a New York City exercise instructor and creator of a fitness lifestyle program called "In Fitness and In Health," suggests the following stretches for this stressed-out area of the body. (Since these exercises are not as unobtrusive as those in remedy 37, you might want to wait until you're at home or in a private place to do them.)

- **Lunge:** From a standing position, with your feet together and toes pointing forward, "lunge" forward with your right foot. Keep your knees bent and your chest up as you lunge. Be sure your right heel strikes the floor before the rest of the foot. And be sure that you keep your right knee aligned above your right ankle; do not bend your right knee so far that it extends forward beyond the ankle. Return to the normal standing position. Repeat 11 more times; then lunge 12 times with the left foot. To increase the intensity of this stretch, do lunges onto a step or small platform.

- **Tendon Stretch:** Stand with both feet on a step or a phone book, with your heels extending beyond the edge of the step. You may want to hold onto something to keep your balance as you shift your weight toward your heels and gently stretch the muscles and tendons in the back of your lower leg.

- **Towel Lift:** Sit on the floor with your legs extended in front of you. Bend your left knee, and put your left foot flat on the floor. Place a towel around your right ankle. Grasping the ends of the towel, use it to pull your right leg up. Keep your right leg straight, and keep your buttocks on the floor as you do so. Hold the stretch for several seconds; then lower your leg to the floor. Repeat with the left leg.

- **"V" Stretch:** Sit on the floor and place your legs out in front of you in a "V" shape. Turn your torso to the right and place your hands on the floor—one hand on either side of your right thigh. Roll your left hip and your left toes inward, so that the inside of your left foot is resting on the floor and the toes of your left foot are pointing toward your right leg. You should feel a stretch in the inner side of your left thigh. Release the stretch, and then repeat the exercise in the opposite direction, with your hands next to your left thigh and your torso turned to the left.

- **Knee Hug:** Sit on the floor with your legs out in front of you. Cross your right leg over your left, with your right knee bent. Hug your right leg to your chest. After putting your right leg back on the floor, cross your left leg over and repeat the hug.

- **Quad Stretch:** Stand behind a chair with your left hand on the back of the chair to help you maintain your balance. Bend your right knee, raise your right foot up behind you, and grasp the right foot with your right hand. Gently pull upward on the foot until it reaches the buttocks. Hold it there for several seconds. You should feel a stretch in the large muscle at the front of your thigh. (Do not arch your back as you do this exercise.) Place your right foot back on the floor, and repeat the stretch with the left foot.

- **Crouch:** Stand in front of a stable chair and hold your arms straight out in front of you (parallel to the floor). Gradually begin to sit down—but stop before your buttocks touch the chair. Your weight should be on your heels; your arms should help you maintain your balance. Stand up again slowly and repeat. Rest, then do another two sets.

- **Towel Scrunch:** Sit on a chair and place your bare feet on the floor. Pretend you have a towel under your toes; draw the towel in toward your heels by scrunching your toes. Then reverse the exercise by using your toes to push the imaginary towel out and away from the heel. Do this ten times with each foot.

- **Towel Scoop:** Sit on a chair and place your bare feet on the floor. Use the outer part of your foot to scoop the imaginary towel in toward your arches. Then use the inner part of your foot to smooth the towel back out. Do this ten times with each foot.

39

WALK, DON'T RUN.

Years ago, no one thought of walking as "real" exercise. Now we know that it's not just a good workout—it's one of the best fitness activities for the feet and for the whole body. As recently as July of 1993, several national health organizations—including the Centers for Disease Control and the President's Council on Physical Fitness and Sports—issued fitness guidelines praising the benefits of moderate exercise and specifically recommending walking.

First, however, it's important to say a few words about running—what most people used to think of as "real" exercise—and the feet. If you're a runner, with each stride you take, you place pressure on the joints of your foot equal to three to four times your normal body weight. That's quite a shock even for healthy feet. For people who already have bone or joint problems, running is even more harmful. And the impact of your feet pounding the pavement intensifies the pressure your shoes exert on problems such as bunions, hammertoes, corns, injured toenails, or bruised heels.

Walking aids weight loss: An average-weight person burns close to 100 calories a mile, about the same amount per mile you would burn running. Your metabolism, or calorie burning, not only speeds up during the time you're actually walking; your body continues to burn fat at a higher-than-usual rate for up to six hours after you have completed your workout.

But walking improves your overall health in an even more important way. If you do it briskly (at a rate of between three and five miles per hour) and continuously for at least 20 to 30 minutes, it becomes an aerobic exercise. An exercise is aerobic if you can do it rhythmically and continuously and at a brisk enough pace to force your heart and lungs to work harder to supply your major muscles with oxygen. By forcing your cardiovascular system to pump blood and oxygen continuously throughout your body, aerobic exercise stimulates and strengthens the heart, lungs, and muscles. It also promotes circulation and, when done on a regular basis, helps to control blood-cholesterol levels, which in turn can help keep your arteries clear and healthy. (The result is that, by engaging in a regular aerobic exercise program, you'll be less likely to suffer from high blood pressure, heart disease, or heart attack. A landmark 20-year study completed in 1989 showed that people who briskly walked two miles a day cut their risk of heart attack by about 28 percent.)

There's more: A walking routine can help you stop smoking; it reduces the craving for nicotine and helps to counteract the sluggish feeling many people have when they first give up cigarettes. It can improve your lung capacity, which is especially important for asthmatics, and can even help to relieve constipation. (Asthmatics and other individuals with significant health problems should be sure to talk to their doctor before beginning any exercise program; see the precautions in remedy 40.) Some studies have even indicated that a fitness-walking program can play a part in helping prevent certain types of cancer.

But in addition to all these great incentives, regular walking is good specifically for your feet. It strengthens the foot muscles and conditions them so that if you do subject them to unusual strain, they're less likely to be injured or ache afterward. Because walking continuously moves joints without placing them under great pressure, it is often recommended as a good way for people with foot-joint problems, including arthritis, gout, and bunions, to get some exercise. Also, because walking is what's called a "weight-bearing exercise"—the demands of the exercise are increased by gravity because you're toting around your own weight—it strengthens the bones in your feet, lessening the chance of fracture and helping to prevent severe bone problems such as osteoporosis. As mentioned earlier, a study at Washington University in St. Louis showed that postmenopausal women actually increased their bone mass through a regular walking routine.

40

BEGIN ANY FITNESS PROGRAM GRADUALLY.

A walking program, or any other fitness program, should be embarked upon gradually, especially if you've never been very active. Plunging head first—or feet first—into a long, vigorous walk after months or years of inactivity will result not in fitness or weight loss, but pain. Begin a walking routine very modestly and, over weeks and months, slowly increase its intensity. You might start out by walking for 20 minutes a day, three days a week, and gradually add to both the length and frequency of your walks so that, after the first three or four months, you are walking for 45 minutes a day, five days a week. The latter schedule—at a pace of at least three miles an hour—should produce aerobic benefits. But even if you can never walk this far or this fast, you will still improve the strength of foot muscles and bones (and your overall health) by walking.

To prevent injury, be sure to do stretches and other light exercises (such as those suggested in remedy 38) before and after your walk; the organizations listed in remedy 50 can send you instructions for other "warm-up" and "cool-down" techniques, as well as information on how to pace yourself.

There are three main styles of walking: slow (nonaerobic) walking, fitness (aerobic) walking, and something called racewalking, which is that funny-looking style you've seen at the Olympics. Racewalking is, indeed, a sport—characterized by straight legs (no bending at the knees), swiveling hips, pumping arms bent at the elbows, and speeds as high as seven or eight miles an hour. It should be attempted only by people who are already in very good physical condition. You do not, however, need to become a racewalker to achieve fitness through walking. And if you are an average fitness walker, you don't need to use wrist and ankle weights while you walk in order to increase the difficulty of your workouts. They're not necessary for aerobic fitness, and if your bones and muscles can't hold up under the added strain, you may create new injuries and other lasting problems for yourself.

Even veteran walkers can sometimes overdo it. While you're out walking, pay attention to the signals your body is sending you. You should never be so short of breath that you can't hold a conversation. If you feel pain in any part of your foot or leg, stop—you may have strained a muscle or injured yourself in some other way, or you may be becoming dehydrated and need fluids.

To decrease the likelihood that you will overdo a walking routine on impulse—and to increase your chances of getting help for injuries if you do—walk with a partner or join a walking club. To find out if there's a club in your area, call your local YMCA or YWCA, inquire at health clubs, or look for notices posted in schools, libraries, and grocery stores. Many shopping malls also sponsor walking groups that walk inside the mall either before the stores open or after they close.

A few final cautions on exercise—*consult a doctor first if you:*

- are older than 50 and not accustomed to regular exercise

- are significantly overweight

- have a history of heart trouble or high blood pressure

- have arthritis or another bone or joint problem

- have a medical condition, such as diabetes, that needs everyday attention

- are on a prescription drug that might interfere with perspiration.

Many such people are actually among those who can benefit most from walking—but a doctor should help them choose the length and intensity of their walking routines.

41

LOSE EXCESS WEIGHT AND CHANGE BAD EATING HABITS.

The heavier you are, the more weight you place on your feet. When you stand, your feet must support your body weight. When you walk, the pressure increases to one-and-a-half times that amount because, as you take each step, most of your weight is shifted onto the front foot. Most people walk between seven and ten miles a day just in the course of their daily activities.

If you have foot problems that hurt under pressure—such as corns, very tough calluses, a bunion, a hammertoe, a bruised or cracked heel, a neuroma, or a heel spur—you have an extra incentive to relieve some of the burden on your feet by losing weight. Other problems, such as certain nail problems, can be the direct result of poor nutrition, so if you start a weight-loss program that's based on good nutrition, you'll help alleviate those foot woes as well.

Dieting and exercise are complementary partners in a successful weight-loss program—and, of course, exercise is another way to strengthen feet and ward off problems. If you exercise without changing your eating habits, you'll lose weight, but it will take much longer. All by itself, a regular walking routine—say, three miles a day, five days a week—will result in only about half a pound of weight loss per week. If you modify your diet but don't exercise, you'll also lose weight, but about a third of the weight you lose will come from muscle rather than fat.

If you're not clearly "overweight," how can you tell if you should shed some pounds? Take the "pinch test": Put your hands on the sides of your hips and "pinch" out the extra flesh. Every quarter inch of flab stands for ten pounds you could lose. A doctor can also help you decide if—and how—you should lose weight.

42

PROVIDE SPECIAL FOOT RELIEF IF YOU MUST STAND FOR LONG PERIODS OF TIME.

Sometimes you simply can't get off your feet, because your job requires you to stand or walk a lot or because you're stuck in an area where there isn't a place to sit down. In the latter situation—for instance, if you're sightseeing or shopping all day—do whatever you can to temporarily relieve the pressure on each foot. Walk as much as you can rather than stand still; wiggle your toes; shift back and forth from one foot to another; stand on one foot while lifting the other slightly off the ground and rotating the ankle.

If you do a lot of walking or standing on the job, keep two pairs of shoes at the office, one with a medium heel and one pair of flats—then switch back and forth throughout the day. Each pair of shoes will require you to use a different set of foot muscles, so this way your whole foot will get exercise. (You'll also relieve the pressure that each pair may exert on different parts of your feet, helping to prevent calluses and corns and relieving bunion pain.) Make sure both pairs of shoes, however, are comfortable; a single hour of standing still in uncomfortable shoes can cause your feet more soreness than a full day's worth of walking in comfortable shoes.

If you stand in one spot throughout your workday, bring in a piece of carpet to stand on (standing on carpet helps to lessen the strain on foot and leg muscles). Periodically slip off your shoes, raise yourself up on tiptoe and come back down again, flex each foot, and wiggle your toes.

While you're standing for several hours, your feet can swell by as much as ten percent. So whenever you do finally get a chance to sit down, try to prop your feet up on something. Elevating them above the level of your hips, even if only for a little while, will help them return to their normal size.

43

MMMMMMM....MASSAGE YOUR FEET.

Throughout this book, foot massage has been mentioned as a remedy for many types of foot pain, from sudden cramps to the ongoing aches of pregnancy. But here's a little secret: Massage also makes your feet healthier. The stronger and more limber your foot muscles are, the less likely they are to feel tired or to sustain injury. And it's a key recovery tool for those who have recently had foot surgery: By drawing more blood to the feet, massage helps speed healing.

Before any foot massage, relax your foot muscles by warming them up. You can do this simply with a heating pad. Or you might prefer a soak in warm water and Epsom salts for about 15 minutes. A third option: Hold your feet under running water for ten minutes while you gradually increase, and then gradually decrease, its temperature (be careful not to let the water get too hot). Another option is the special towel wrap described in remedy 5.

Now you're ready to begin the massage. Prop one foot up on the other leg's knee and turn the sole toward you. Spread moisturizing lotion or cream on the sole of the foot or on your hands. Using your thumbs, massage the soles in a deep, circular motion. Start at the area just behind your toes and work backward to the heel. Concentrate your efforts on one small area at a time. When you've covered the entire sole, turn your foot over and massage the top, still using your thumbs. Again, work on one spot at a time and cover the whole top of the foot. After that, it's time to turn your attention to your toes. Give each one a slow, gentle tug; massage it by twisting its sides, working from the base of the toe outward; then wiggle it back and forth. Now repeat the same procedure on the other foot.

Although the above routine will give you a good general massage, here are some little tricks that will further increase circulation and give your feet a tingling feeling:

- Pinch along the outside edges of your foot.

- Lightly slap the soles with the back of your hand or gently pound the sole with a relaxed fist; follow this with a stroking motion along the length of the sole.

- Use both hands to twist the foot in opposite directions, wringing it like a sponge.

- If one spot on your foot is tight and aches, instead of massaging it, just press down hard on the spot with your thumbs, hold for several seconds, then release.

You might also try using a cream or rub that contains menthol during your foot massage for a refreshing touch. Finally, if your feet need rubbing but you don't want to or you can't do it yourself because of arthritis or some other medical condition, you might want to try a foot whirlpool device that will massage your feet for you. (You should avoid strong vibrations, however, if you have a history of blood clots.) These whirlpool devices can usually be purchased in drugstores.

44

KNOW YOUR REAL SHOE SIZE (AND WIDTH AND HEEL HEIGHT).

As mentioned earlier, one person can have two feet that are slightly different in size and shape. And even if yours seem identically matched, they don't necessarily remain a constant size. Your feet can actually be different sizes at different times of the day. There are also more lasting changes: Most feet gradually widen with age, and sometimes women's feet "grow" (because of muscle relaxation during pregnancy) after the birth of a child.

Shop for shoes in the late afternoon or evening, since that's when your feet are the biggest (they swell during the day). Have the salesperson measure both feet while you're standing up, since your feet expand under the weight of your body. Carefully consider the fit and walking comfort of each pair of shoes you try and keep in mind that "size 8" in three different styles, even from the same manufacturer, can fit your feet differently.

If you have wide feet, always ask (even if the salesperson has measured your feet) if the style you've chosen comes in a wide width. Fortunately, comfortable shoes have become popular—even stylish—and shoe manufacturers are waking up to the fact that not everyone has a medium-width foot. Some manufacturers make shoes as wide as triple-E (on a scale of A to E, with AAAA being the narrowest).

There are two other contributors to your shoe "size" as well: The *shape* of your foot (how the shoe's "upper" conforms to your foot) and the heel height that is best for you. Since high heels shift body weight onto the front of your feet, heavy people and people with bunions, corns, hammertoes, and the like should opt for lower heels. If you have excessively pronated ("flat") feet, Achilles tendinitis, short calf muscles, or knee problems, however, shoes with a moderate heel may be more comfortable, since they lessen the pull on already-overstretched tendons and muscles.

45

WALK RIGHT PAST THESE KILLER SHOE STYLES.

Give your feet a break and avoid the six foot-foiling shoe styles discussed here:

- *A stiletto heel* or any other heel that is higher than three inches redistributes your body weight so that 90 percent of it is on the front of your feet. This can create calluses; increase the pain of bunions, hammertoes, and corns; and strain muscles and tendons. They also make maintaining your balance quite a challenge.

- *Pointy-toe shoes* squeeze the toes together, causing uncomfortable calluses and corns. Pointy shoes can also put pressure on ingrown toenails and bunions and increase the likelihood of hammertoes.

- *Flats* can be a problem not just for people with arch and Achilles-tendon problems, but for anyone who wears them exclusively. Over time, your foot gets used to being pronated (flattened), and you may develop arch pain and tendinitis. Alternate flats with shoes that have a moderate heel.

- *Mules* generally have a high heel, and so you're likely to have all the same problems as those mentioned above, when too much pressure is placed on the front of the foot. In addition, the lack of heel support increases your chance of injury if your foot turns on the heel or slips out of the shoe.

- *Platform shoes,* popular in the 1970s, have unfortunately come back in style in the '90s. Like high heels, they are so unstable that you can't help but periodically turn your ankle, possibly causing muscle strain, a sprain, or a fracture.

- *Old shoes* with worn-down heels or traction, flattened insoles, stretched-out uppers, or unraveling stitching can cause you to slip, can strain foot muscles, and can lead to ankle sprains.

46

GET THE SUPPORT YOU NEED FROM SHOES.

Most people think that trying on shoes is about how the shoes feel on your feet. That's true. Certainly, if they don't feel good, you don't want them. But you should evaluate shoes on several more specific factors:

- The toe box should be roomy enough for your toes to rest comfortably. Too much room can allow feet to slide inside shoes, causing calluses and other irritation. The more common problem is that the toe box is too tight. There should also be room in front of the toes, at least ⅜ to ½ inch between your longest toe and the front of the shoe when you are standing. And there should be room above your toes to prevent the shoe from rubbing against them, causing corns. To test the above criteria, make sure you can wiggle your toes inside the toe box when standing.

- A shoe's "upper"—the material on the top of it—should conform to the shape of your foot. It should provide support but also "give" when your foot moves. Look for an upper made of a material that is nonirritating and porous, allowing air into the shoe. Leather is more likely than vinyl to have these characteristics. (Polish leather shoes frequently to help the uppers stay soft and supple.)

- The shoe should provide ample cushioning to absorb shock on foot bones and muscles each time you take a step. You need such cushioning in three key areas: the arch; the front, where the ball of the foot rests; and the heel, which normally supports 25 percent of your body weight. If the insole material is also absorbent, it will help relieve heat inside shoes and prevent rashes and the spread of infection.

- Soles should provide adequate traction to prevent slipping on any surfaces where you expect to be wearing the shoes.

- Heels should ideally provide slight elevation (between ¾ and 1 inch) for the foot, whether there's an actual heel or a sole that's thicker toward the back of the shoe. The counter—the part that curves around the back of your heel—should be stiff enough to prevent ankle strains and sprains. The back of your foot should fit snugly into the heel of the shoe.

Two more general tips: If your two feet are different sizes, choose shoes that fit the bigger foot. (You can pad or add support inserts to the other shoe.) And never buy shoes that are too stiff or too tight with the expectation that you will "break them in": You're likely to suffer much longer than you expected.

Although all this means that you must be a sophisticated and patient shoe shopper, the good news is that many fashionable shoes currently on the market meet all of these qualifications, and many even resemble athletic shoes in design (see remedy 47). This is especially good news for the 59 percent of American women who wear high-heeled shoes every day. As consumers have become more health conscious, shoe manufacturers have given new attention to developing good-looking shoes (even with heels) that won't hurt your feet.

47

BE PICKY IN CHOOSING ATHLETIC SHOES.

When you choose sport or fitness shoes, you are looking for the same attributes as with regular shoes: good traction; cushioning inside the shoe; a soft, porous upper; a firm, snug-fitting heel; a roomy toe box; and overall comfort. But while these qualities are preferable in regular shoes, they are essential in athletic shoes; the absence of any one can cause pain and even injury.

Running shoes tend to have especially good traction to prevent slipping, as well as very thick soles to soften the blow delivered to your feet every time they land hard on the ground. You need those features for running. You don't need them for a walking routine, although you do need a shoe that's sturdier than most sneakers or tennis shoes. Fortunately, because walking has become such a popular fitness exercise in recent years, you can now find a large selection of walking shoes in most shoe and department stores. In addition to following the same shoe-shopping guidelines given in remedies 44 and 46, consider these tips specifically for choosing walking shoes:

- The upper of a good walking shoe will be sturdier than that of a regular shoe but more flexible than that of a running shoe. This is necessary because a walking stride requires more foot flexibility than a running stride.

- The depth of the shoe's tread should also be greater than that of a regular shoe but less than that of a running shoe, in order to provide the traction necessary for a smooth yet stable walking stride. One reason not to do a walking routine in running shoes is that the traction of the latter is so deep it can make you jam your feet (causing toe injuries) and even stumble while walking. Also, the thick soles and stiff uppers of running shoes can make them too heavy for walking.

- Shoes that have a reinforced toe will help prevent toe injuries and help the toe box of the shoe remain sturdy longer. Most walking shoes will have a slightly raised toe, which helps your foot move more comfortably in the conventional "rocking" motion of a walking stride.

- Don't assume that you'll buy walking shoes in the same size as your everyday shoes. Take into account the thickness of the sock you expect to wear while walking (and you should wear thick, absorbent socks). It is best to bring the socks along and put them on when you are trying on walking shoes. This way, you won't have to guess at how much room to leave for the socks. Also, remember that your feet will probably swell as you walk. It may be helpful to do some actual walking around before you shop for the shoes, to give your feet a chance to swell a bit.

- A porous upper and an absorbent inner lining are essential in helping to prevent rashes and infection. They can also help your feet to stay cooler, drier, and more comfortable as you walk. You might also want to look for shoes that have a removable, absorbent insole to keep your feet dry.

- The sole area under the heel should be slightly thicker than it is under the rest of the shoe, elevating your heel ½ to ¾ inch above the ball of your foot; this elevation will help prevent tendon and arch strain. Make sure that the heel "collar" (the part above the heel counter) is firm fitting but well padded to prevent blisters and that the insole under the heel is well padded. Inner-heel padding is especially important on a street or sidewalk.

- Keep in mind that if you plan to do a lot of walking on uneven, rocky terrain, you will need walking shoes that provide more protection and stability. Ask the salesperson to point out styles designed for trail and off-trail walkers.

- Worn-down shoes are a simple but common cause of pain and injury. So no matter what type of shoes you wear or activity you do, if you exercise regularly, it's a good idea to buy new athletic shoes every four to six months or whenever the tread wears down.

48

BE A SMART SHOPPER WHEN BUYING FOOT-CARE PRODUCTS.

Here's the bottom line on most of the foot-care products you'll find on the market today:

For foot comfort and support: Some insoles offer only a thin, generically shaped cushion of support, while others are designed to fit a particular shoe style or to provide extra support or padding in specific areas. As styles vary, though, so does price: In one major drugstore chain, insoles cost anywhere from 99 cents to $8.99 a pair. Other items you can purchase include specially shaped padding to place around bunions, corns, and hurt toes; lamb's wool or moleskin to fashion your own padding; foam arch-support inserts and heel pads; and rubber heel cups.

For calluses: The only callus products that really help get rid of thick, painful calluses—and that are safe—are cushioning products, pumice stones or other buffing products, footbath products, and moisturizing creams. Skip the "callus removers" (medicated pads) and "callus trimmers." The former contain salicylic acid, which can burn not just the callused area but more sensitive skin around it, and the latter actually has a blade (you should never cut a callus).

For corns: "Corn removers" also contain salicylic acid, but since corns are generally more painful than calluses, many people prefer to remove them with these liquids, creams, or medicated pads. If you use them, first place doughnut-shaped padding around the corn to protect the surrounding skin. "Corn files"—to file away the corn as you would file your nails—are rarely effective.

For ingrown toenails: Over-the-counter products don't actually change the position or growth of the nail; they just temporarily stop the pain by softening the skin around the nail while it grows out. An antiseptic applied daily helps prevent infection, which is the biggest danger with an ingrown nail.

For warts: Wart-remover solutions and medicated pads contain salicylic acid and are quite effective in making warts disappear—but use them very carefully so that you don't apply the treatment to healthy skin. If you're applying a solution, put a doughnut-shaped pad or petroleum jelly around the wart to protect healthy skin.

For athlete's foot and other fungal infections: Here you'll find probably the widest selection of brand names in a variety of formulations. While the ingredients in these products vary somewhat, most of them contain tolnaftate or undecylenate. Look for one that also contains silicone powder to absorb moisture.

For dry skin: Most moisturizing creams contain the same ingredients: vegetable oils, mineral oils, and lanolin. You can also buy soaps or footbath products with ingredients that not only soften but also disinfect your feet. To treat scaly, itchy, dry skin, look for products with 10% lactic acid.

For sunburn: If your feet sunburn easily (and most do), try using a "sports" sunscreen, which should have a sun protection factor (SPF) of at least 15. The sunscreen you choose should also be waterproof, in case your feet get wet.

49

KNOW WHEN NOT TO TREAT YOURSELF—AND HOW TO FIND THE BEST DOCTOR.

When you use this book to look up a particular foot problem, read the section carefully, because with almost any problem there are some circumstances in which certain individuals, such as people with diabetes or circulation problems, should see a doctor rather than attempting to self-treat. Likewise, if you are under the continuing care of a physician for any reason or have recently had surgery, discuss your foot pain with your doctor.

Some foot problems should never be treated with home remedies; always seek medical attention for the following:

- fracture

- foreign body embedded in the foot

- severe ankle sprain

- dog, snake, or other animal bite

- pinched nerve

- psoriasis or other serious skin disorder

- deformities of children's feet, such as club foot or webbed or overlapping toes

- foot problems that occur in conjunction with a serious disease (for instance, Kaposi's sarcoma, or skin lesions often associated with HIV)

- any lump inside the foot that appears mysteriously (which could be a tumor)

- unexplained pain, swelling, and tenderness around a bone (which could be a sign of osteomyelitis, a very serious bone infection, or osteosarcoma, bone cancer).

Aside from these specific situations, your best general guidelines as to when to see a doctor are the extent and the duration of your discomfort. Extreme pain is a sign that something is seriously wrong; even if you believe you know how to treat it, you should consult an expert. And if you follow the advice given for your problem and it still doesn't go away—if pain, itching, swelling, discoloration, or any other symptom of the problem persists—see a podiatrist.

Podiatrists—doctors who specialize in diagnosing and treating foot problems—have the letters D.P.M., which stands for Doctor of Podiatric Medicine, after their name. Some podiatrists have a narrower focus in their practice, treating just sports injuries to the foot; for information about this specialty, write to the American Academy of Podiatric Sports Medicine (the address is listed in remedy 50). When choosing a podiatrist, you will want to consider the same factors you do in choosing any other doctor. Try to speak with other patients to find out about their experiences. When you meet the doctor for the first time, ask as many questions as you need to in order to feel that he or she understands your problem. Also, ask about hospital affiliations and experience in treating your particular problem. To locate a board-certified podiatrist in your area, ask for recommendations from a major hospital, your state department of health, or the American Podiatric Medical Association. The latter has a toll-free hotline, 800-FOOTCARE.

STAY EDUCATED AND INFORMED ABOUT FOOT CARE.

The following organizations can give you additional, free information.

SPECIFIC PROBLEMS AND GENERAL FOOT HEALTH

American Podiatric Medical Assn.
9312 Old Georgetown Rd.
Bethesda, MD 20814-1621
800-FOOTCARE

American Orthopedic Foot
and Ankle Society
701 16th Ave.
Seattle, WA 98122
800-235-4855

American College of Foot
and Ankle Surgeons
444 N. Northwest Hwy., #150
Park Ridge, IL 60068-3263
800-421-2237

American College of Foot Orthopedics
and Medicine
4603 Hwy. 95 South, Box 39
Cocolalla, ID 83813-0039
208-683-3900

CARE OF AGING
AND ARTHRITIC FEET

National Institute on Aging
NIA Information Center
Box 8057
Gaithersburg, MD 20898-8057

American Assn. of Retired Persons
601 "E" St. NW
Washington, DC 20049

Arthritis Foundation
Box 19000
Atlanta, GA 30326
800-283-7800

WALKING AND OTHER EXERCISE

American Heart Assn.
7272 Greenville Ave.
Dallas, TX 75231
800-AHA-USA1

President's Council on Physical
  Fitness and Sports
701 Pennsylvania Ave. NW, #250
Washington, DC 20004

Rockport Walking Institute
Box 30
Marlborough, MA 01752
800-343-WALK

American Academy of Podiatric
  Sports Medicine
1729 Glastonberry Rd.
Potomac, MD 20854

INDEX